CANCER-FIGHTING

BLENDS

A Comprehensive Anti-Cancer Smoothie Cookbook

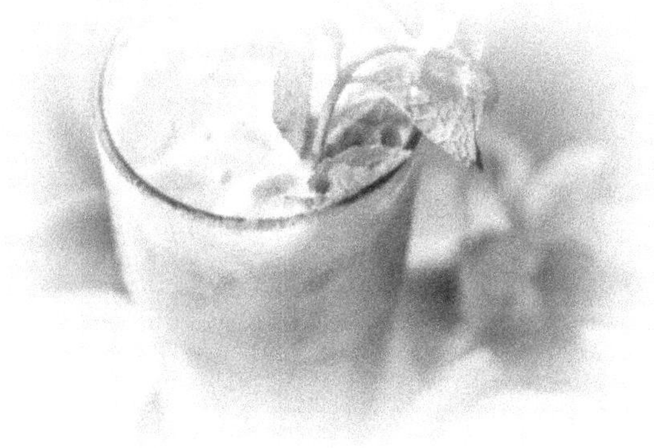

MARRIES-ESTHER LLOYD

TABLE OF CONTENT

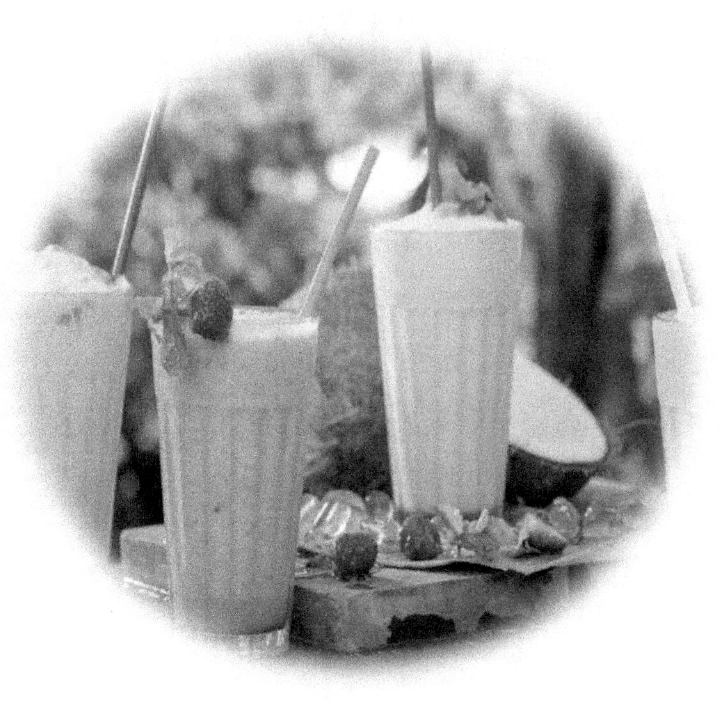

INTRODUCTION

In the bustling city of New York years ago, amidst the towering skyscrapers and bustling streets, lived Esther, a vibrant soul with a spirit as resilient as the city itself. Yet, beneath her seemingly ordinary exterior, Esther carried a burden that would test her strength in ways she never imagined. Diagnosed with cancer, she faced a daunting journey filled with uncertainty and fear.

Determined to fight with every ounce of her being, Esther embarked on a quest for healing that would lead her down unexpected paths. Amidst the sea of treatments and therapies, she stumbled upon a beacon of hope – anti-cancer smoothies.

Intrigued by the idea of harnessing the power of nature's bounty to combat the disease ravaging her body, Esther delved into the world of cancer-fighting blends with unwavering determination.

Armed with a blender and an arsenal of nutrient-rich ingredients, Esther embarked on a daily ritual of blending vibrant fruits, vegetables, and super foods into delicious concoctions that not only nourished her body but also fuelled her fight against cancer. With each sip of these potent elixirs, she felt a surge of vitality course through her veins, empowering her to face each day with renewed vigour and optimism.

As weeks turned into months, Esther's journey took a remarkable turn. Against all odds, she witnessed first-hand the transformative power of anti-cancer smoothies as her health began to improve, and the tumour that once loomed menacingly began to shrink.

With each passing day, Esther grew stronger, her spirit buoyed by the tangible evidence of her body's remarkable ability to heal itself.

Inspired by her own miraculous journey, Esther felt compelled to share her newfound knowledge and passion for cancer-fighting blends with the world. And thus, "Cancer-Fighting Blends: A Comprehensive Anti-Cancer Smoothie Cookbook" was born – a labour of love dedicated to empowering others on their path to healing.

Dear reader, within the pages of this book, lies a treasure trove of recipes, insights, and guidance to help you harness the healing power of anti-cancer smoothies. Whether you're battling cancer yourself or seeking to support a loved one on their journey to wellness, this cookbook offers a beacon of hope and a roadmap to vibrant health.

Join Esther and countless others who have experienced the life-changing benefits of anti-cancer smoothies. Together, let us embark on a journey of healing, resilience, and hope. Let this book be your guide as you harness the transformative power of nature's bounty to fight back against cancer and reclaim your health and vitality.

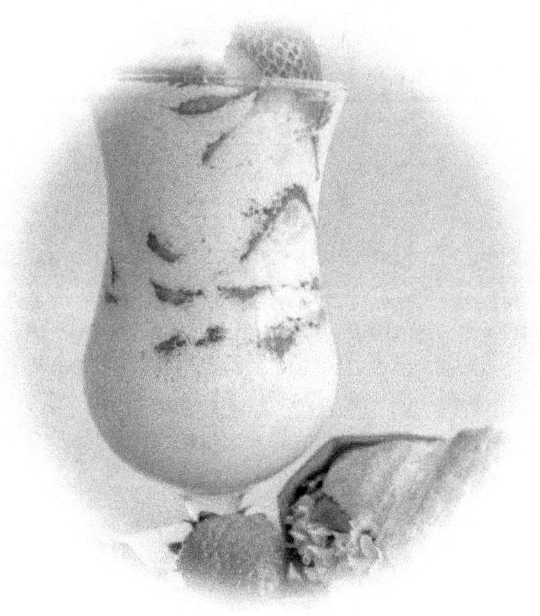

CHAPTER 1

INTRODUCTION TO CANCER-FIGHTING NUTRITION

In the quest for a healthy lifestyle, the significance of nutrition cannot be emphasized enough. As we delve into the intricate web of our well-being, it becomes increasingly evident that the food we consume plays a pivotal role in shaping our health outcomes.

This is especially true in the context of cancer prevention, where emerging research underscores the profound impact of a nutrient-rich diet on mitigating the risk of this formidable adversary.

The Link between Nutrition and Cancer Prevention

Scientific studies have illuminated a compelling link between nutrition and the prevention of cancer. While genetics and environmental factors certainly contribute, our dietary choices have a profound influence on the body's ability to ward off potential threats.

Consuming a diverse array of nutrient-dense foods has been associated with bolstering the immune system, reducing inflammation, and maintaining optimal cellular function — all of which are crucial elements in the defence against cancer.

By understanding and embracing the power of food as medicine, we can actively engage in practices that promote overall health and resilience.

Through this cookbook, we aim to unravel the mysteries of cancer-fighting nutrition, empowering you to make informed choices that not only tantalize the taste buds but also fortify your body against the onset of cancer.

Explanation of Key Nutrients and Antioxidants Found in Fruits, Vegetables, and Other Ingredients

Nature has endowed us with a cornucopia of foods rich in key nutrients and antioxidants that exhibit potent anti-cancer properties. From vibrant fruits like berries, bursting with cancer-fighting phytochemicals, to cruciferous vegetables such as broccoli and kale, known for their detoxifying prowess, our culinary palette is replete with ingredients designed to promote health at the cellular level.

In this cookbook, we will delve into the specifics of these nutritional powerhouses, elucidating the role of vitamins, minerals, and antioxidants in preventing cellular damage, inhibiting the growth of cancer cells, and supporting the body's natural defence mechanisms.

By understanding the science behind these nutrients, you will be better equipped to make informed choices and craft smoothies that serve as a potent ally in your quest for well-being.

Introduction to the Concept of Using Smoothies

Recognizing the challenges of modern life, we present an innovative and delectable solution to seamlessly integrate these cancer-fighting ingredients into your daily routine: The Anti-Cancer Smoothie.

Beyond a mere beverage, a well-crafted smoothie becomes a delightful canvas upon which you can artfully blend a symphony of flavours and health benefits.

Smoothies offer a convenient and delicious way to transform a medley of anti-cancer foods into a single, palatable concoction. Whether you are a seasoned wellness enthusiast or just embarking on your journey to a healthier lifestyle, the recipes in this cookbook will guide you in harnessing the inherent power of nutrition, one sip at a time.

 Join us in this culinary adventure as we embark on a journey to nourish the body and fortify the spirit against the challenges that lie ahead.

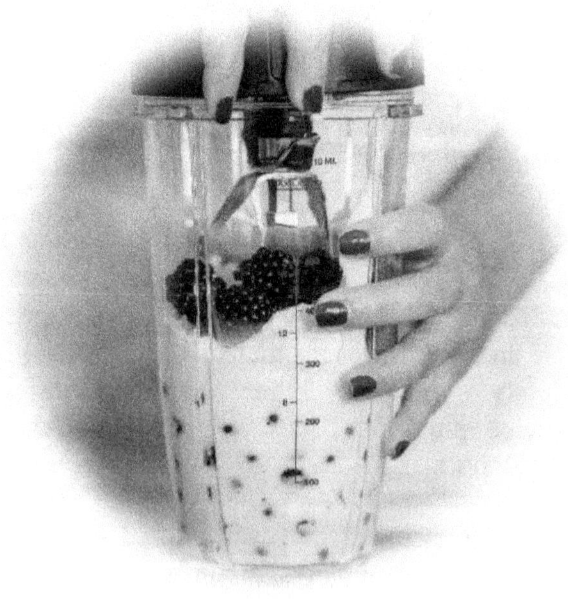

CHAPTER 2

BUILDING THE FOUNDATION - ESSENTIAL INGREDIENTS

In the quest for crafting potent anti-cancer smoothies, it's imperative to build a solid foundation grounded in the selection of key ingredients. This chapter is dedicated to exploring and understanding the intricacies of these essential components, each chosen for its remarkable anti-cancer properties and nutritional prowess.

Detailed Profiles of Superfoods

Berries:

Berries, such as blueberries, strawberries, and raspberries, emerge as veritable superstars in the anti-cancer arena. Rich in antioxidants, specifically flavonoids and polyphenols, these tiny treasures have demonstrated the ability to neutralize free radicals, reducing oxidative stress and the risk of cellular damage.

Anthocyanins, the compounds responsible for the vibrant hues of berries, have been linked to inhibiting the growth of cancer cells and supporting overall cellular health.

Leafy Greens:

The verdant family of leafy greens, including kale, spinach, and Swiss chard, contributes an array of essential nutrients. Packed with vitamins A, C, and K, as well as minerals like iron and calcium, leafy greens offer a nutritional powerhouse that supports immune function, promotes detoxification, and fosters optimal cell division.

Furthermore, they contain chlorophyll, known for its potential in preventing carcinogenesis and enhancing the body's ability to eliminate toxins.

Turmeric:

Celebrated for its vibrant golden hue and centuries-old medicinal use, turmeric contains curcumin, a potent anti-inflammatory compound with promising anti-cancer properties.

Curcumin has been shown to interfere with various stages of cancer development, including inhibiting the proliferation of cancer cells and impeding the formation of blood vessels that nourish tumours.

Incorporating turmeric into your smoothies not only adds a delightful earthy flavour but also infuses your concoction with a powerful anti-cancer punch.

Ginger:

Renowned for its zesty kick and medicinal attributes, ginger boasts anti-inflammatory and antioxidant properties that may contribute to cancer prevention.

Studies suggest that ginger may impede the growth of cancer cells, induce apoptosis (programmed cell death), and mitigate the side effects of conventional cancer treatments.

Adding a knob of fresh ginger to your smoothies not only enhances flavour but also harnesses its potential anti-cancer benefits.

Tips on Selecting and Preparing Fresh, Organic Ingredients

Selecting high-quality, fresh, and organic ingredients is paramount to maximizing the nutritional benefits of your anti-cancer smoothies. Here are some practical tips:

1. *Choose Organic Produce:* Opt for organic fruits and vegetables to minimize exposure to pesticides and other harmful chemicals. Organic produce is cultivated using environmentally friendly practices that promote soil health and reduce the risk of contamination.

2. *Embrace Seasonality:* Incorporate seasonal produce to ensure freshness and peak nutritional content. Seasonal fruits and vegetables are not only more flavourful but also tend to be more affordable and environmentally sustainable.

3. *Inspect for Quality:* When selecting fruits and vegetables, inspect them for firmness, vibrant colours, and minimal bruising. Fresh, high-quality ingredients contribute to a more palatable and nutritious smoothie.

4. *Proper Storage:* Store ingredients properly to preserve their freshness. Refrigerate perishable items, and keep fruits and vegetables in separate bins to prevent premature ripening.

5. *Prep with Care:* Wash and prep ingredients just before use to retain their nutritional integrity. Consider leaving skins on fruits and vegetables when appropriate, as they often contain valuable nutrients.

Information on the Nutritional Benefits of Each Ingredient

Understanding the nutritional benefits of each ingredient is crucial for tailoring your smoothies to specific health goals. This section provides insights into how these superfoods contribute to cancer prevention:

- *Antioxidants:* Berries and leafy greens are rich in antioxidants that combat oxidative stress, reducing the risk of DNA damage and cell mutations associated with cancer.

- *Anti-Inflammatory* Properties: Turmeric and ginger possess anti-inflammatory compounds that may help inhibit the inflammatory processes linked to cancer development.

- *Vitamins and Minerals:* Leafy greens provide essential vitamins (A, C, K) and minerals (iron, calcium) crucial for immune function, DNA repair, and overall cellular health.

- *Curcumin in Turmeric:* Curcumin in turmeric has shown promise in inhibiting the growth of cancer cells and preventing the formation of blood vessels that support tumours.

- *Ginger's Bioactive Compounds:* Ginger's bioactive compounds, including gingerol, have demonstrated anti-cancer effects by inducing apoptosis and inhibiting the growth and spread of cancer cells.

By comprehending the unique contributions of each ingredient, you can craft smoothies that not only tantalize your taste buds but also provide a robust defence against cancer, one sip at a time.

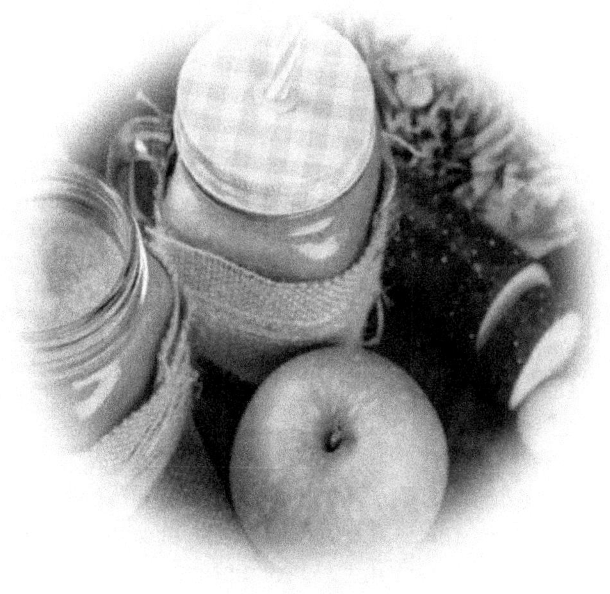

CHAPTER 3

TAILORING SMOOTHIES FOR SPECIFIC CANCERS

Addressing the nuances of individual health needs is paramount in the pursuit of cancer prevention and support. In this chapter, we delve into the art of tailoring anti-cancer smoothies to cater to specific types of cancers.

Through customized recipes, evidence-based nutritional advice, and adaptive strategies, we aim to empower individuals with tools to proactively contribute to their well-being.

Customized Recipes and Nutritional Advice

Understanding that different cancers may have distinct nutritional requirements, this section provides tailored recipes and nutritional guidance for specific types of cancers. Each recipe is meticulously crafted to include ingredients that have demonstrated potential benefits in scientific studies.

Prostate Cancer:

- *Ingredients*: Incorporate tomatoes (rich in lycopene), green tea (high in antioxidants), and flaxseeds (source of omega-3 fatty acids).

- *Nutritional Focus*: Emphasize foods rich in lycopene, selenium, and zinc, which have been associated with prostate health. Consider the inclusion of green tea for its potential anti-cancer properties.

Breast Cancer:

- *Ingredients*: Include cruciferous vegetables (e.g., broccoli, cauliflower), berries, and green leafy vegetables.

- *Nutritional Focus*: Emphasize foods rich in phytoestrogens, such as flaxseeds and soy, which may have protective effects. Incorporate cruciferous vegetables known for their potential anti-cancer properties.

Lung Cancer:

- Ingredients: Integrate ginger, turmeric, and dark green leafy vegetables.

- Nutritional Focus: Emphasize foods with anti-inflammatory and antioxidant properties, such as ginger and turmeric. Dark green leafy vegetables provide essential vitamins and minerals for lung health.

These customized recipes serve as a starting point, offering a flavourful and nutrient-rich approach tailored to specific cancer types. However, it is crucial to consult with healthcare professionals for personalized advice and to ensure compatibility with ongoing treatments.

Incorporating Ingredients from Scientific Studies

Scientific studies continue to shed light on the potential benefits of specific ingredients in the context of cancer prevention and support. By incorporating these findings into our recipes, we aim to provide a foundation rooted in evidence-based nutrition.

Example: **Lung Cancer:**

- *Ingredient*: Green tea extract

- *Scientific Rationale*: Studies suggest that green tea polyphenols may have anti-cancer effects, particularly in reducing the risk of lung cancer. Incorporating green tea extract into smoothies offers a concentrated source of these beneficial compounds.

Example: **Breast Cancer:**

- *Ingredient*: Pomegranate seeds

- Scientific Rationale: Research indicates that pomegranate extracts may inhibit the growth of breast cancer cells. Including pomegranate seeds in smoothies provides a delicious and potentially beneficial addition.

By staying informed about the latest scientific findings, individuals can make proactive choices in crafting smoothies that align with their health goals and may contribute to cancer prevention.

Guidance on Adapting Recipes to Meet Individual Dietary Needs and Preferences

Recognizing the diverse dietary needs and preferences of individuals, this section offers guidance on adapting anti-cancer smoothie recipes to accommodate various lifestyles.

1. *Allergies and Sensitivities*: Provide alternative ingredients for common allergens, ensuring that individuals with dietary restrictions can still enjoy the benefits of anti-cancer smoothies.

2. *Texture and Consistency*: Offer variations in recipes to accommodate preferences for thicker or thinner smoothies, allowing individuals to tailor the texture to their liking.

3. *Flavour Profiles*: Suggest ingredient substitutions or additions to cater to diverse taste preferences, ensuring that individuals find the smoothies enjoyable and palatable.

4. *Customization Tips*: Encourage experimentation with ingredient quantities, allowing individuals to adjust flavours and nutritional profiles according to personal preferences.

By offering flexibility and adaptability in the recipes, this cookbook aims to empower individuals to integrate anti-cancer smoothies into their lifestyles in a way that aligns with their unique dietary needs and tastes.

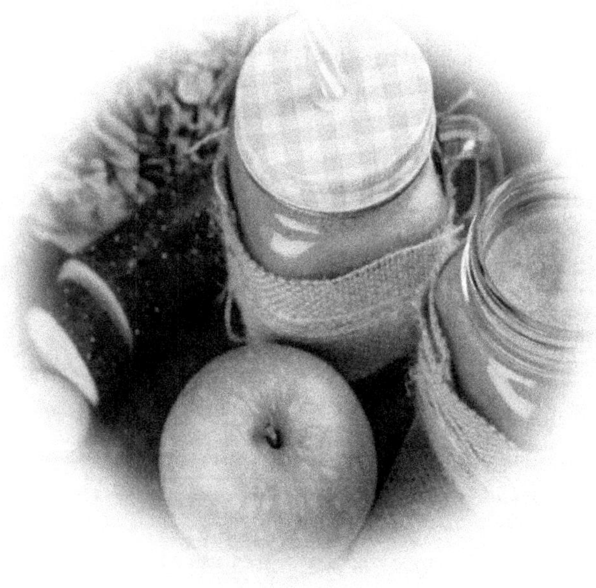

CHAPTER 4

ANTI-CANCER SMOOTHIES RECIPES

Here are 60 anti-cancer smoothie recipes, along with their ingredients and methods of preparation:

1. **Berry Bliss Smoothie**
   - *Ingredients:*
   - 1 cup of assorted berries, including strawberries, blueberries, and raspberries.
      - 1 banana
      - 1 cup spinach
      - 1 cup almond milk
      - Ice cubes (optional)

   - *Method:* Blend all the components until they form a smooth mixture.

2. **Tropical Turmeric Delight**
   - *Ingredients:*
      - 1 cup pineapple chunks
      - 1/2 cup mango
      - 1 teaspoon turmeric powder
      - 1 cup coconut milk
      - Ice cubes (optional)

   - *Method:* Blend all ingredients until well combined.

3. **Green Goddess Elixir**
   - *Ingredients:*
     - Handful of kale leaves
     - 1/2 cucumber
     - 1 green apple
     - Fresh mint leaves
     - 1 cup water or coconut water

   - *Method:* Blend all the components until they form a smooth mixture.

4. **Citrus Surge Smoothie**
   - *Ingredients:*
     - 2 oranges, peeled and segmented
     - 1 grapefruit, peeled and segmented
     - 1 teaspoon grated ginger
     - 1 cup water
     - Ice cubes (optional)

   - *Method:* Blend all ingredients until a refreshing smoothie is achieved.

5. **Creamy Avocado Dream**
   - *Ingredients:*
     - 1 ripe avocado
     - 1 banana
     - 1 cup almond milk
     - Honey to taste
     - Ice cubes (optional)
   - *Method:* Blend all ingredients until creamy and well-blended.

6. **Superseed Power Smoothie**
   - *Ingredients:*
       - 2 tablespoons chia seeds
       - 1 tablespoon flaxseeds
       - 1 cup mixed berries
       - 1 banana
       - 1 cup Greek yogurt
       - 1 cup water or almond milk

   - *Method:* Blend until seeds are well incorporated.

7. **Restorative Berry Chamomile Blend**
   - *Ingredients:*
       - 1 cup chamomile tea, cooled
       - 1/2 cup mixed berries
       - 1 tablespoon honey
       - Ice cubes (optional)

   - *Method:* Brew chamomile tea and let it cool. Blend with berries and honey.

8. **Turmeric Sunshine Citrus Splash**
   - *Ingredients:*
       - 1 teaspoon turmeric powder
       - 1 orange, peeled and segmented
       - 1/2 lemon, juiced
       - 1 cup water
       - Ice cubes (optional)
   - *Method:* Blend until a vibrant, citrusy smoothie is achieved.

9. Pomegranate Paradise
  - *Ingredients:*
    - 1/2 cup pomegranate seeds
    - 1 cup mixed berries
    - 1 banana
    - 1 cup coconut water
    - Ice cubes (optional)

  - *Method:* Blend until a refreshing pomegranate-infused smoothie is obtained.

10. Ginger Zinger Green Smoothie
  - *Ingredients:*
    - 1 inch fresh ginger, peeled
    - Handful of spinach
    - 1 green apple, cored
    - 1/2 cucumber
    - 1 cup water or coconut water

  - *Method:* Blend until the ginger adds a zesty kick to this green concoction.

11. Cranberry Citrus Crush
  - *Ingredients:*
    - 1/2 cup cranberries (fresh or unsweetened dried)
    - 1 orange, peeled and segmented
    - 1/2 cup Greek yogurt
    - 1 cup water or almond milk
  - *Method*: Blend until a tangy and antioxidant-rich smoothie is achieved

12. **Blue Almond Bliss**
 - *Ingredients:*
    - 1 cup blueberries
    - 1/2 cup almonds, soaked
    - 1 banana
    - 1 cup almond milk
    - Ice cubes (optional)

 - *Method:* Blend until the almonds contribute to a creamy texture.

13. **Minty Melon Magic**
 - *Ingredients:*
    - 1 cup watermelon, cubed
    - 1/2 cup cucumber
    - Fresh mint leaves
    - 1 tablespoon lime juice
    - Ice cubes (optional)

 - *Method:* Blend until a refreshing and hydrating smoothie is achieved.

14. **Beet Berry Boost**
 - *Ingredients:*
    - 1 small beetroot, boiled and peeled.
    - 1 cup mixed berries
    - 1 banana
    - 1 cup water or coconut water

 - *Method:* Blend until the vibrant colour and earthy sweetness of beets infuse the smoothie.

15. **Carrot Ginger Energizer**
   - *Ingredients:*
      - 1 cup carrot juice
      - 1 inch fresh ginger, peeled
      - 1 orange, peeled and segmented
      - Ice cubes (optional)

   - *Method:* Blend until a zingy and nutrient-packed smoothie is achieved.

16. **Spinach Pineapple Paradise**
   - *Ingredients:*
      - Handful of spinach
      - 1 cup pineapple chunks
      - 1 banana
      - 1 cup coconut water
      - Ice cubes (optional)

   - *Method:* Blend until the sweetness of pineapple complements the earthiness of spinach.

17. **Cinnamon Apple Pie Smoothie**
   - *Ingredients:*
      - 1 apple, cored and sliced
      - 1/2 teaspoon cinnamon
      - 1/2 cup oats (cooked and cooled)
      - 1 cup almond milk
      - Ice cubes (optional)

   - *Method:* Blend until reminiscent of the comforting flavours of apple pie.

18. **Kiwi Kale Crush**
  - *Ingredients:*
    - 2 kiwis, peeled and sliced
    - Handful of kale leaves
    - 1 banana
    - 1 cup water or coconut water

  - *Method:* Blend until the tartness of kiwi blends harmoniously with the nutrient-rich kale.

19. **Anti-Inflammatory Golden Elixir**
  - *Ingredients:*
    - 1 teaspoon turmeric powder
    - 1/2 teaspoon cinnamon
    - 1/4 teaspoon black pepper (to enhance turmeric absorption)
    - 1 cup coconut milk
    - Honey to taste

  - *Method:* Blend until a golden elixir with anti-inflammatory properties is achieved.

20. **Mango Basil Bliss**
  - *Ingredients:*
    - 1 cup mango chunks
    - Fresh basil leaves
    - 1 banana
    - 1 cup water or coconut water
    - Ice cubes (optional)
  - *Method:* Blend until the tropical sweetness of mango melds with the aromatic freshness of basil.

21. **Strawberry Shortcake Smoothie**
- Ingredients:
1 cup strawberries, hulled
1/2 cup oats (cooked and cooled)
1 banana
1 cup almond milk
Ice cubes (optional)

Method: Blend all the ingredients until smooth and creamy.

22. **Raspberry Almond Radiance**
- Ingredients:
  - 1 cup raspberries
  - 1/2 cup almonds, soaked
  - 1 banana
  - 1 cup almond milk
  - Ice cubes (optional)

- *Method:* Blend until the richness of almonds complements the tartness of raspberries.

23. **Mango Turmeric Tango**
- Ingredients:
  - 1 cup mango chunks
  - 1 teaspoon turmeric powder
  - 1/2 teaspoon ginger, grated
  - 1 cup coconut water
  - Ice cubes (optional)
- *Method:* Blend until the tropical sweetness of mango dances with the warmth of turmeric.

24. **Cocoa Berry Antioxidant Delight**
  - *Ingredients:*
      - 1 cup mixed berries
      - 1 tablespoon cocoa powder (unsweetened)
      - 1 banana
      - 1 cup almond milk
      - Ice cubes (optional)

  - *Method:* Blend until the rich antioxidants of berries meet the decadence of cocoa.

25. **Papaya Paradise**
  - *Ingredients:*
      - 1 cup papaya chunks
      - 1/2 cup pineapple chunks
      - 1 banana
      - 1 cup coconut water
      - Ice cubes (optional)

  - *Method:* Blend until the tropical sweetness of papaya transports you to paradise.

26. **Peachy Keen Kale Kick**
  - *Ingredients:*
      - 1 peach, pitted and sliced
      - Handful of kale leaves
      - 1 banana
      - 1 cup water or almond milk

  - *Method:* Blend until the velvety sweetness of peaches meets the robustness of kale.

27. **Blueberry Basil Bliss**
  - *Ingredients:*
    - 1 cup blueberries
    - Fresh basil leaves
    - 1 banana
    - 1 cup coconut water
    - Ice cubes (optional)

  - *Method:* Blend until the aromatic essence of basil elevates the sweetness of blueberries.

28. **Fig and Walnut Wonder**
  - *Ingredients:*
    - 1/2 cup dried figs, soaked
    - 1/4 cup walnuts
    - 1 banana
    - 1 cup almond milk
    - Ice cubes (optional)

  - *Method:* Blend until the natural sweetness of figs pairs with the nutty crunch of walnuts.

29. **Acai Berry Burst**
  - *Ingredients:*
    - 1 packet frozen acai puree
    - 1/2 cup mixed berries
    - 1 banana
    - 1 cup coconut water
    - Ice cubes (optional)

- *Method:* Blend until the superfood acai combines with a medley of berries for a burst of antioxidants.

30. **Apricot Almond Ambrosia**
  - *Ingredients:*
    - 1 cup apricots, pitted and sliced
    - 1/2 cup almonds, soaked
    - 1 banana
    - 1 cup almond milk
    - Ice cubes (optional)

  - *Method:* Blend until the delicate sweetness of apricots intertwines with the creaminess of almonds.

31. **Cranberry Kale Kick-start**
  - *Ingredients:*
    - 1/2 cup cranberries (fresh or unsweetened dried)
    - Handful of kale leaves
    - 1 green apple, cored
    - 1 cup water or coconut water

  - *Method:* Blend until the tartness of cranberries kicks up the nutrient-packed kale.

32. **Orange Carrot Crush**
  - *Ingredients:*
    - 2 oranges, peeled and segmented
    - 1 cup carrot juice
    - 1/2 inch ginger, grated
    - Ice cubes (optional)

  - *Method:* Blend until the citrusy zing of oranges complements the earthy sweetness of carrots.

33. **Pumpkin Spice Delight**
  - *Ingredients:*
    - 1/2 cup canned pumpkin puree
    - 1/2 teaspoon pumpkin spice blend
    - 1 banana
    - 1 cup almond milk
    - Ice cubes (optional)

  - *Method:* Blend until the warm spices of pumpkin spice create a delightful autumnal treat.

34. **Cherry Almond Amour**
  - *Ingredients:*
    - 1 cup cherries, pitted
    - 1/2 cup almonds, soaked
    - 1 banana
    - 1 cup almond milk
    - Ice cubes (optional)
  - *Method:* Blend until the sweet-tart flavour of cherries mingles with the creamy richness of almonds.

35. **Matcha Green Zen**
  - *Ingredients:*
     - 1 teaspoon matcha powder
     - Handful of spinach
     - 1 banana
     - 1 cup coconut water
     - Ice cubes (optional)

  - *Method:* Blend until the vibrant green of matcha meets the nourishing essence of spinach.

36. **Mint Chocolate Euphoria**
  - *Ingredients:*
     - Handful of fresh mint leaves
     - 1 tablespoon cocoa powder (unsweetened)
     - 1 banana
     - 1 cup almond milk
     - Ice cubes (optional)

  - *Method:* Blend until the cooling sensation of mint harmonizes with the indulgence of cocoa.

37. **Dragon Fruit Extravaganza**
  - *Ingredients:*
     - 1 cup dragon fruit, cubed
     - 1/2 cup strawberries
     - 1 banana
     - 1 cup coconut water
     - Ice cubes (optional)
  - *Method:* Blend until the vibrant pink of dragon fruit creates an exotic and visually stunning smoothie.

38. **Hazelnut Fig Fantasy**
  - *Ingredients:*
    - 1/2 cup dried figs, soaked
    - 1/4 cup hazelnuts
    - 1 banana
    - 1 cup almond milk
    - Ice cubes (optional)

  - *Method:* Blend until the natural sweetness of figs meets the nutty allure of hazelnuts.

39. **Watermelon Mint Refresher**
  - *Ingredients:*
    - 2 cups watermelon, cubed
    - Fresh mint leaves
    - 1 tablespoon lime juice
    - Ice cubes (optional)

  - *Method:* Blend until the hydrating essence of watermelon combines with the invigorating notes of mint.

40. **Lemon Ginger Zest**
  - *Ingredients:*
    - 1 lemon, peeled and segmented
    - 1/2 inch ginger, grated
    - 1 banana
    - 1 cup water or coconut water
    - Ice cubes (optional)

  - *Method:* Blend until the zesty brightness of lemon intertwines with the warmth of ginger.

41. **Raspberry Rose Elixir**
 - *Ingredients:*
    - 1 cup raspberries
    - 1/2 cup rose water
    - 1 banana
    - 1 cup almond milk
    - Ice cubes (optional)

 - *Method:* Blend until the delicate floral notes of rose water complement the sweetness of raspberries.

42. **Blackberry Basil Breeze**
 - *Ingredients:*
    - 1 cup blackberries
    - Fresh basil leaves
    - 1 banana
    - 1 cup coconut water
    - Ice cubes (optional)
 - *Method*: Blend until the aromatic basil adds a refreshing twist to the rich flavour of blackberries.

43. **Cucumber Mint Cooler**
 - *Ingredients:*
    - 1/2 cucumber
    - Fresh mint leaves
    - 1 green apple, cored
    - 1 cup water or coconut water

 - *Method:* Blend until the hydrating cucumber mingles with the cooling essence of mint.

44. Golden Mango Turmeric

  - *Ingredients:*
    - 1 cup mango chunks
    - 1 teaspoon turmeric powder
    - 1/2 teaspoon cinnamon
    - 1 cup coconut water
    - Ice cubes (optional)

  - *Method*: Blend until the vibrant gold of turmeric blends with the tropical sweetness of mango.

45. Blueberry Basil Bliss

  - *Ingredients:*
    - 1 cup blueberries
    - Fresh basil leaves
    - 1 banana
    - 1 cup coconut water
    - Ice cubes (optional)

  - *Method:* Blend until the aromatic essence of basil elevates the sweetness of blueberries.

46. Cinnamon Apple Pie Smoothie

  - *Ingredients:*
    - 1 apple, cored and sliced
    - 1/2 teaspoon cinnamon
    - 1/2 cup oats (cooked and cooled)
    - 1 cup almond milk
    - Ice cubes (optional)

  - *Method:* Blend until reminiscent of the comforting flavours of apple pie.

47. **Kiwi Kale Crush**
- *Ingredients:*
    - 2 kiwis, peeled and sliced
    - Handful of kale leaves
    - 1 banana
    - 1 cup water or coconut water
- *Method*: Blend until the tartness of kiwi melds with the nutrient-rich kale.

48. **Anti-Inflammatory Golden Elixir**
- *Ingredients:*
    - 1 teaspoon turmeric powder
    - 1/2 teaspoon cinnamon
    - 1/4 teaspoon black pepper (to enhance turmeric absorption)
    - 1 cup coconut milk
    - Honey to taste

- *Method:* Blend until a golden elixir with anti-inflammatory properties is achieved.

49. **Mango Basil Bliss**
- *Ingredients:*
    - 1 cup mango chunks
    - Fresh basil leaves
    - 1 banana
    - 1 cup water or coconut water
    - Ice cubes (optional)

- *Method*: Blend until the tropical sweetness of mango melds with the aromatic freshness of basil.

50. **Strawberry Shortcake Smoothie**
- *Ingredients:*
    - 1 cup strawberries, hulled
    - 1/2 cup oats (cooked and cooled)
    - 1 banana
    - 1 cup almond milk
    - Ice cubes (optional)

- *Method*: Blend until oats contribute to a creamy texture reminiscent of strawberry shortcake.

51. **Dragon Fruit Extravaganza**
- *Ingredients:*
    - 1 cup dragon fruit, cubed
    - 1/2 cup strawberries
    - 1 banana
    - 1 cup coconut water
    - Ice cubes (optional)

- *Method*: Blend until the vibrant pink of dragon fruit creates an exotic and visually stunning smoothie.

52. **Hazelnut Fig Fantasy**
- *Ingredients:*
    - 1/2 cup dried figs, soaked
    - 1/4 cup hazelnuts
    - 1 banana
    - 1 cup almond milk
    - Ice cubes (optional)

- *Method*: Blend until the natural sweetness of figs meets the nutty allure of hazelnuts.

53. **Watermelon Mint Refresher**
- *Ingredients:*
    - 2 cups watermelon, cubed
    - Fresh mint leaves
    - 1 tablespoon lime juice
    - Ice cubes (optional)

- *Method*: Blend until the hydrating essence of watermelon combines with the invigorating notes of mint.

54. **Lemon Ginger Zest**
- *Ingredients:*
    - 1 lemon, peeled and segmented
    - 1/2 inch ginger, grated
    - 1 banana
    - 1 cup water or coconut water
    - Ice cubes (optional)
- *Method*: Blend until the zesty brightness of lemon intertwines with the warmth of ginger.

55. **Raspberry Rose Elixir**
  - *Ingredients*:
    - 1 cup raspberries
    - 1/2 cup rose water
    - 1 banana
    - 1 cup almond milk
    - Ice cubes (optional)

  - *Method*: Blend until the delicate floral notes of rose water complement the sweetness of raspberries.

56. **Blackberry Basil Breeze**
  - *Ingredients*:
    - 1 cup blackberries
    - Fresh basil leaves
    - 1 banana
    - 1 cup coconut water
    - Ice cubes (optional)

  - *Method*: Blend until the aromatic basil adds a refreshing twist to the rich flavour of blackberries.

57. **Cucumber Mint Cooler**
  - *Ingredients*:
    - 1/2 cucumber
    - Fresh mint leaves
    - 1 green apple, cored
    - 1 cup water or coconut water

  - *Method*: Blend until the hydrating cucumber mingles with the cooling essence of mint.

58. **Golden Mango Turmeric**
- *Ingredients:*
    - 1 cup mango chunks
    - 1 teaspoon turmeric powder
    - 1/2 teaspoon cinnamon
    - 1 cup coconut water
    - Ice cubes (optional)

- *Method:* Blend until the vibrant gold of turmeric blends with the tropical sweetness of mango.

59. **Blueberry Basil Bliss**
- *Ingredients:*
    - 1 cup blueberries
    - Fresh basil leaves
    - 1 banana
    - 1 cup coconut water
    - Ice cubes (optional)

- *Method*: Blend until the aromatic essence of basil elevates the sweetness of blueberries.

60. **Cinnamon Apple Pie Smoothie**
- *Ingredients*:
    - 1 apple, cored and sliced
    - 1/2 teaspoon cinnamon
    - 1/2 cup oats (cooked and cooled)
    - 1 cup almond milk
    - Ice cubes (optional)

- *Method*: Blend until reminiscent of the comforting flavours of apple pie.

Enjoy these additional anti-cancer smoothie recipes, each packed with delicious flavours and health-boosting ingredients!

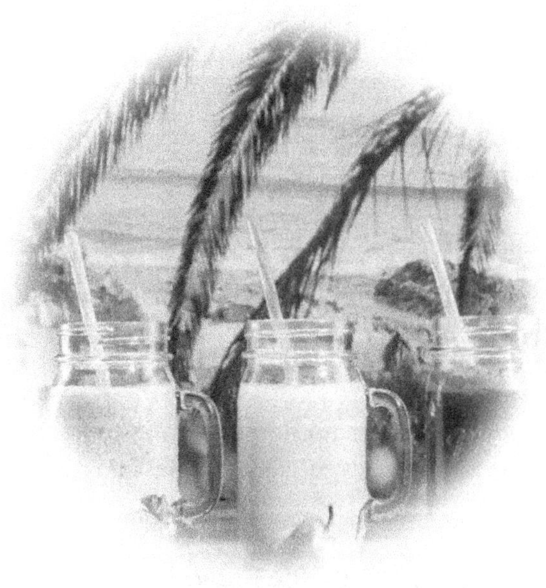

Chapter 5

30-DAY ANTI-CANCER SMOOTHIE CHALLENGE

Embark on a transformative journey with our 30-Day Anti-Cancer Smoothie Challenge. This section provides a structured plan featuring diverse, delicious smoothie recipes, daily motivation tips, and tools to track your progress.

As you sip your way through this challenge, you'll not only tantalize your taste buds but also cultivate habits that contribute to your overall well-being.

A 30-Day Plan Featuring a Variety of Delicious Smoothie Recipes

Diversity is the key to sustained health benefits. Our 30-day plan introduces an array of delectable smoothie recipes, each crafted to provide a unique combination of anti-cancer ingredients.

From the vibrant hues of berry blends to the earthy richness of turmeric-infused creations, this plan ensures a delightful and nutritious experience every day.

Example Week:

1. *Berry Bliss Monday:* A refreshing blend of blueberries, strawberries, and spinach.

2. *Tropical Turmeric Tuesday:* Pineapple, mango, turmeric, and coconut milk create a zesty and anti-inflammatory concoction.

3. *Green Goddess Wednesday:* Kale, cucumber, green apple, and mint unite for a detoxifying and nutrient-packed smoothie.

4. *Citrus Surge Thursday:* Oranges, grapefruit, and a touch of ginger for a citrusy burst of vitamin C and antioxidants.

5. *Creamy Avocado Friday:* Avocado, banana, and almond milk create a creamy, heart-healthy smoothie.

6. *Superseed Saturday:* Chia seeds, flaxseeds, and berries for a fibre and omega-3 fatty acid boost.

7. *Restorative Sunday:* A soothing blend of chamomile tea, honey, and berries for relaxation and antioxidants.

This diverse selection ensures that participants enjoy a spectrum of flavours and nutritional benefits throughout the challenge.

Daily Tips and Encouragement to Help Readers Stay Motivated

Staying motivated is key to successfully completing the 30-day challenge. Each day, participants receive tips and encouragement to keep them inspired and engaged. These daily prompts may include:

1. Educational Nuggets: Brief insights into the nutritional benefits of the day's featured ingredients, fostering a deeper understanding of their anti-cancer properties.

2. Wellness Wisdom: Practical advice on incorporating healthy habits beyond smoothies, such as staying hydrated, getting sufficient sleep, and engaging in physical activity.

3. Community Connection: Encouragement to share experiences, photos, and thoughts on social media platforms using a designated hashtag, fostering a sense of community and accountability.

4. Mindful Moments: Reminders to practice mindfulness and savour the sensory experience of

each smoothie, cultivating a mindful approach to eating.

5. Celebrate Milestones: Acknowledgment of achievements at the end of each week, reinforcing the positive impact of the challenge on overall well-being.

Tracking Tools and Journal Prompts to Monitor Impact on Health

To enhance self-awareness and monitor progress, participants are provided with tracking tools and journal prompts. These include:

1. *Daily Log:* A simple tracker to record the smoothie consumed, physical activity, sleep quality, and overall mood each day.

2. *Reflection Journal:* Weekly prompts encouraging participants to reflect on changes in energy levels, cravings, and any noticeable improvements in well-being.

3. *Goal Setting:* Encouragement to set personal health goals and revisit them throughout the challenge, adapting them as needed.

4. *Gratitude Journal:* A space to express gratitude for the nourishing foods and positive habits

cultivated during the challenge, fostering a positive mind set.

By incorporating these elements, the 30-Day Anti-Cancer Smoothie Challenge becomes more than just a culinary adventure. It becomes a holistic journey toward better health, providing participants with the tools, motivation, and awareness to make lasting changes for a vibrant and resilient future.

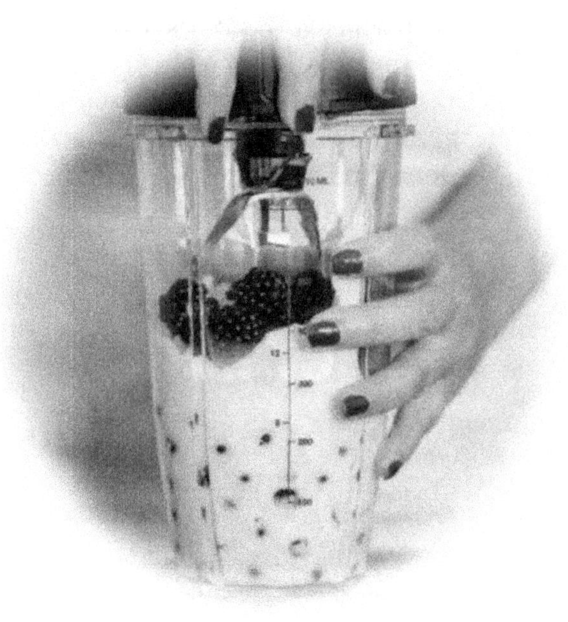

Chapter 6

LIFESTYLE TIPS FOR CANCER PREVENTION

Cancer prevention extends beyond the contents of a glass; it encompasses a comprehensive approach to daily living. This chapter delves into lifestyle tips that complement the anti-cancer smoothies, fostering a holistic environment for well-being.

Beyond Smoothies: Exploring a Holistic Approach to Cancer Prevention

Cancer prevention is not a one-size-fits-all endeavour; it requires a multifaceted approach. Beyond the delightful concoctions of anti-cancer smoothies, consider incorporating the following elements into your lifestyle:

1. Regular Physical Activity:

   - Engage in regular exercise to promote overall health and reduce the risk of certain cancers.

   - Choose activities that you enjoy, making it more likely to become a sustainable part of your routine.

2. Stress Management:

   - Engage in activities that alleviate stress, such as meditation, yoga, or deep breathing exercises.

   - Chronic stress can impact the immune system, and finding effective ways to manage stress contributes to overall well-being.

3. Adequate Sleep:

   - Make quality sleep a priority, targeting 7-9 hours per night.

   - Quality sleep is crucial for the body's repair processes, immune function, and overall resilience.

4. Tobacco and Alcohol Moderation:

   - If applicable, avoid or quit smoking, and limit alcohol consumption.

   - Both tobacco and excessive alcohol use are linked to an increased risk of various cancers.

5. Regular Health Check-ups:

- Arrange routine check-ups and screenings as advised by healthcare professionals.

- Early detection and intervention play a vital role in cancer prevention and treatment.

Lifestyle Habits and Dietary Choices that Complement Anti-Cancer Smoothie Recipes

Optimizing cancer prevention involves aligning dietary choices with healthy lifestyle habits. In tandem with anti-cancer smoothies, consider the following:

1. Hydration:

- Give importance to staying hydrated by consuming a sufficient amount of water throughout the day.

- Staying well-hydrated supports overall bodily functions, aiding in digestion, circulation, and toxin elimination.

2. Balanced Nutrition:

- Maintain a well-balanced diet rich in a variety of fruits, vegetables, whole grains, lean proteins, and healthy fats.

- Diversity in food choices ensures a broad spectrum of nutrients, contributing to overall health.

3. Limit Processed Foods:

- Minimize the consumption of processed and sugary foods, which may contribute to inflammation and other health issues.

- Choose whole, nutrient-rich foods to supply essential vitamins and minerals.

4. Portion Control:

- Practice mindful eating and be conscious of portion sizes to prevent overconsumption.

- Controlling portions helps maintain a healthy weight, reducing the risk of obesity-related cancers.

5. Limit Red and Processed Meats:

- Consider reducing the intake of red and processed meats, which have been associated with an increased risk of certain cancers.

- Explore plant-based protein sources as alternatives.

Practical Tips for Creating a Healthy and Supportive Environment for Overall Well-being

Cultivating a health-supportive environment is integral to cancer prevention. Consider implementing the following practical tips:

1. *Kitchen Organization*:

- Keep a well-organized kitchen to facilitate easy access to fresh ingredients for smoothies and meals.

- A tidy kitchen encourages regular use of wholesome ingredients.

2. *Meal Planning*:

  - Plan meals and snacks in advance to ensure a well-balanced and varied diet.

  - Planning minimizes reliance on convenience foods and supports healthier choices.

3. *Social Support:*

  - Foster a supportive social environment by sharing your health goals with friends and family.

  - Engage in activities that promote well-being together, such as cooking nutritious meals or participating in physical activities.

4. *Mindful Eating Practices*:

  - Cultivate mindful eating habits by relishing every bite and being attuned to signals of hunger and fullness.

  - Mindful eating promotes a healthy relationship with food and encourages conscious dietary choices.

5. *Environmental Awareness*:

- Be conscious of environmental factors that may impact health, such as exposure to pollutants or harmful chemicals.

- Make choices that align with a healthy and sustainable lifestyle.

By intertwining lifestyle tips with the delightful world of anti-cancer smoothies, this cookbook aims to guide readers toward a holistic approach to cancer prevention—one that nourishes not only the body but also the mind and spirit.

Cheers to you!

MARRIES E. LLOYD.

Author

meknatureconcept@gmail.com

Thank you for choosing this book, if you feel this book is valuable, kindly consider leaving us a review on Amazon. Your feedback is critical to me and others looking for help related to the same book.

WEEKLY MEAL PLANNER

<table>
<tr><td rowspan="3">MONDAY</td><td>BREAKFAST</td><td></td></tr>
<tr><td>LUNCH</td><td></td></tr>
<tr><td>DINNER</td><td></td></tr>
<tr><td rowspan="3">MONDAY</td><td>BREAKFAST</td><td></td></tr>
<tr><td>LUNCH</td><td></td></tr>
<tr><td>DINNER</td><td></td></tr>
<tr><td rowspan="3">MONDAY</td><td>BREAKFAST</td><td></td></tr>
<tr><td>LUNCH</td><td></td></tr>
<tr><td>DINNER</td><td></td></tr>
<tr><td rowspan="3">MONDAY</td><td>BREAKFAST</td><td></td></tr>
<tr><td>LUNCH</td><td></td></tr>
<tr><td>DINNER</td><td></td></tr>
<tr><td rowspan="3">MONDAY</td><td>BREAKFAST</td><td></td></tr>
<tr><td>LUNCH</td><td></td></tr>
<tr><td>DINNER</td><td></td></tr>
<tr><td rowspan="3">MONDAY</td><td>BREAKFAST</td><td></td></tr>
<tr><td>LUNCH</td><td></td></tr>
<tr><td>DINNER</td><td></td></tr>
<tr><td rowspan="3">MONDAY</td><td>BREAKFAST</td><td></td></tr>
<tr><td>LUNCH</td><td></td></tr>
<tr><td>DINNER</td><td></td></tr>
</table>

GROCERY LIST

SNACKS

Smoothie

WEEKLY MEAL PLANNER

			GROCERY LIST
MONDAY	BREAKFAST		
	LUNCH		
	DINNER		
MONDAY	BREAKFAST		
	LUNCH		
	DINNER		
MONDAY	BREAKFAST		
	LUNCH		
	DINNER		
MONDAY	BREAKFAST		
	LUNCH		
	DINNER		
MONDAY	BREAKFAST		
	LUNCH		SNACKS
	DINNER		
MONDAY	BREAKFAST		
	LUNCH		
	DINNER		
MONDAY	BREAKFAST		
	LUNCH		
	DINNER		

Smoothie

WEEKLY MEAL PLANNER

MONDAY	BREAKFAST		GROCERY LIST
	LUNCH		
	DINNER		
MONDAY	BREAKFAST		
	LUNCH		
	DINNER		
MONDAY	BREAKFAST		
	LUNCH		
	DINNER		
MONDAY	BREAKFAST		
	LUNCH		
	DINNER		
MONDAY	BREAKFAST		SNACKS
	LUNCH		
	DINNER		
MONDAY	BREAKFAST		
	LUNCH		
	DINNER		
MONDAY	BREAKFAST		
	LUNCH		
	DINNER		

Smoothie

WEEKLY MEAL PLANNER

MONDAY	BREAKFAST	
	LUNCH	
	DINNER	
MONDAY	BREAKFAST	
	LUNCH	
	DINNER	
MONDAY	BREAKFAST	
	LUNCH	
	DINNER	
MONDAY	BREAKFAST	
	LUNCH	
	DINNER	
MONDAY	BREAKFAST	
	LUNCH	
	DINNER	
MONDAY	BREAKFAST	
	LUNCH	
	DINNER	
MONDAY	BREAKFAST	
	LUNCH	
	DINNER	

GROCERY LIST

SNACKS

Smoothie

WEEKLY MEAL PLANNER

MONDAY	BREAKFAST	
	LUNCH	
	DINNER	
MONDAY	BREAKFAST	
	LUNCH	
	DINNER	
MONDAY	BREAKFAST	
	LUNCH	
	DINNER	
MONDAY	BREAKFAST	
	LUNCH	
	DINNER	
MONDAY	BREAKFAST	
	LUNCH	
	DINNER	
MONDAY	BREAKFAST	
	LUNCH	
	DINNER	
MONDAY	BREAKFAST	
	LUNCH	
	DINNER	

GROCERY LIST

SNACKS

Smoothie

WEEKLY MEAL PLANNER

MONDAY	BREAKFAST	
	LUNCH	
	DINNER	
MONDAY	BREAKFAST	
	LUNCH	
	DINNER	
MONDAY	BREAKFAST	
	LUNCH	
	DINNER	
MONDAY	BREAKFAST	
	LUNCH	
	DINNER	
MONDAY	BREAKFAST	
	LUNCH	
	DINNER	
MONDAY	BREAKFAST	
	LUNCH	
	DINNER	
MONDAY	BREAKFAST	
	LUNCH	
	DINNER	

GROCERY LIST

SNACKS

Smoothie

WEEKLY MEAL PLANNER

				GROCERY LIST
MONDAY	BREAKFAST			
	LUNCH			
	DINNER			
MONDAY	BREAKFAST			
	LUNCH			
	DINNER			
MONDAY	BREAKFAST			
	LUNCH			
	DINNER			
MONDAY	BREAKFAST			
	LUNCH			
	DINNER			
MONDAY	BREAKFAST			SNACKS
	LUNCH			
	DINNER			
MONDAY	BREAKFAST			
	LUNCH			
	DINNER			
MONDAY	BREAKFAST			
	LUNCH			
	DINNER			

Smoothie

WEEKLY MEAL PLANNER

MONDAY		
BREAKFAST	
LUNCH	
DINNER	

MONDAY		
BREAKFAST	
LUNCH	
DINNER	

MONDAY		
BREAKFAST	
LUNCH	
DINNER	

MONDAY		
BREAKFAST	
LUNCH	
DINNER	

MONDAY		
BREAKFAST	
LUNCH	
DINNER	

MONDAY		
BREAKFAST	
LUNCH	
DINNER	

MONDAY		
BREAKFAST	
LUNCH	
DINNER	

GROCERY LIST

SNACKS

Smoothie

WEEKLY MEAL PLANNER

MONDAY	BREAKFAST	
	LUNCH	
	DINNER	
MONDAY	BREAKFAST	
	LUNCH	
	DINNER	
MONDAY	BREAKFAST	
	LUNCH	
	DINNER	
MONDAY	BREAKFAST	
	LUNCH	
	DINNER	
MONDAY	BREAKFAST	
	LUNCH	
	DINNER	
MONDAY	BREAKFAST	
	LUNCH	
	DINNER	
MONDAY	BREAKFAST	
	LUNCH	
	DINNER	

GROCERY LIST

SNACKS

Smoothie

WEEKLY MEAL PLANNER

MONDAY		
BREAKFAST	
LUNCH	
DINNER	

GROCERY LIST

MONDAY		
BREAKFAST	
LUNCH	
DINNER	

MONDAY		
BREAKFAST	
LUNCH	
DINNER	

MONDAY		
BREAKFAST	
LUNCH	
DINNER	

MONDAY		
BREAKFAST	
LUNCH	
DINNER	

SNACKS

MONDAY		
BREAKFAST	
LUNCH	
DINNER	

MONDAY		
BREAKFAST	
LUNCH	
DINNER	

Smoothie